C000180687

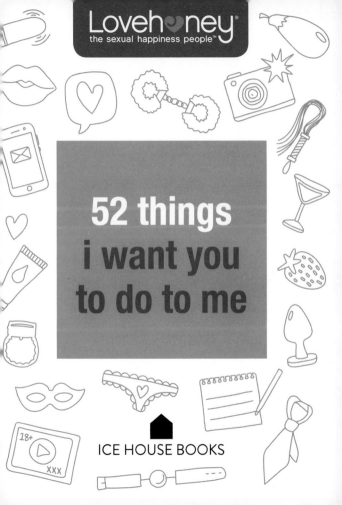

Published by Ice House Books

Copyright © 2020 Lovehoney Group Ltd. Lovehoney® is a
registered trademark of Lovehoney Group Ltd, Bath, BA1 3EN

Ice House Books is an imprint of Half Moon Bay Limited
The Ice House, 124 Walcot Street, Bath, BA1 5BG
www.icehousebooks.co.uk

The material in this publication is of the nature of general
comment only, and does not represent professional advice.

ISBN 978-1-913308-02-5

Printed in China

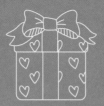

To

From

XOX

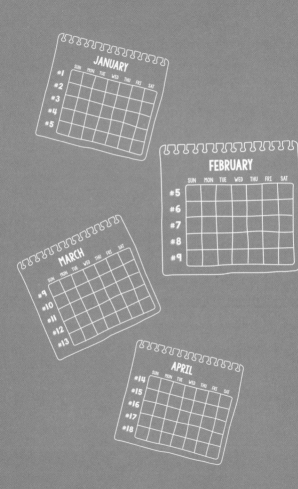

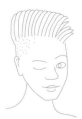
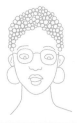
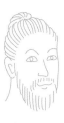

WELCOME

This little book contains **52 things I want you to do to me** – one for every week of the year. Some are romantic, some are raunchy – all are **a whole lot of fun!**

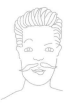
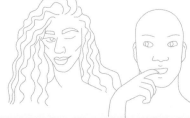

SAFETY & CONSENT

Before embarking on any sort of BDSM journey (Bondage, Domination/Discipline, Sadism/Submission, Masochism), there are some rules you must follow to ensure everything is safe and everyone involved is having fun. At no point should bondage put either person at risk of injury. If something is distractingly painful or uncomfortable, stop immediately, and never leave a restrained person unattended. Ensure that everyone involved is of sound mind. Never explore bondage or spanking while under the influence of drugs or alcohol.

Everything you do together should be 100% consensual. To ensure this is the case, agree a safe word or action before you play.

Safe words or actions are used by partners to indicate that they want play to stop immediately.

Choose a word that is short and easy to remember before play, or try the popular 'traffic light' system, where **'red'** means stop, **'amber'** means take it easy and **'green'** means go on.

If you use a gag, you'll need to agree a safe action instead. Clicking fingers, tapping a hard surface three times or opening and closing your hands repeatedly are popular choices. Avoid using household items that require a knot for first-time bondage. Keep a pair of specially designed safety scissors nearby just in case.

Only share personal photographs or videos of yourself with someone you completely trust. Remember once they are out in the world it's hard to get them back.

#1

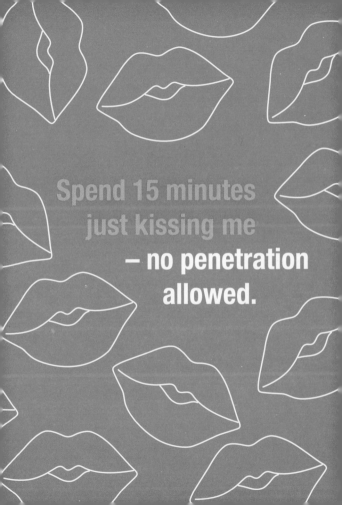

Spend 15 minutes
just kissing me
**– no penetration
allowed.**

#2

Write me a letter
describing
**what you love
about my body.**

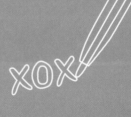

#3

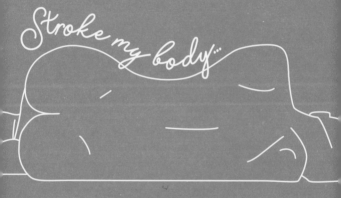

Stroke my body...

all over with a feather
tickler or a soft brush.

#4

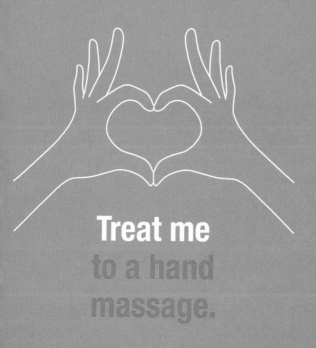

Treat me
to a hand
massage.

#5

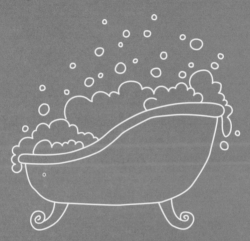

Run a bath for me,
complete with
candles and
bubbles.

#6

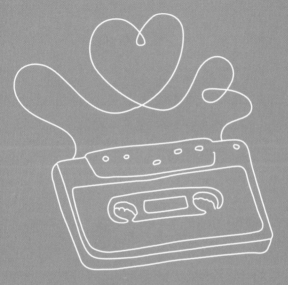

Make a mix tape **(playlist)** of romantic or meaningful songs for me.

#7

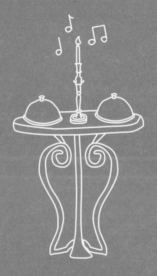

Cook a special meal
I will love, play my
favourite music and
turn the lights down low.

#8

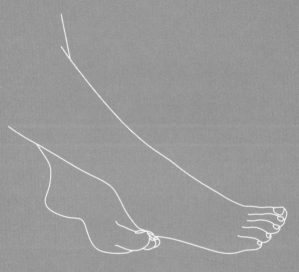

Give me a foot rub for at least five minutes.

#9

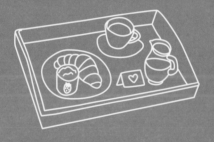

Treat me for the
entire day, starting with
breakfast in bed.

#10

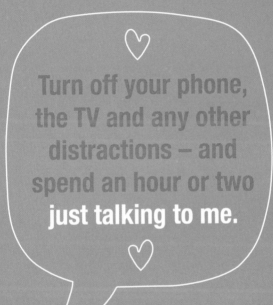

#11

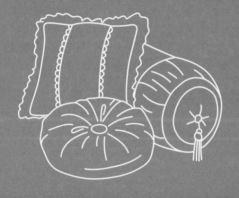

Arrange cushions and blankets on our living room floor and have a **candlelit picnic with me.**

#12

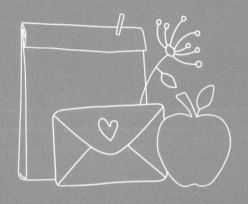

Make me lunch to take
to work and slip in a
love note or **flower.**

#13

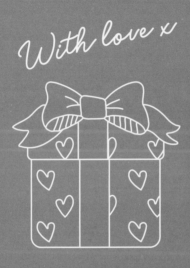

With love x

Buy or make me a little gift
that you know I will like – it
doesn't need to be expensive!

#14

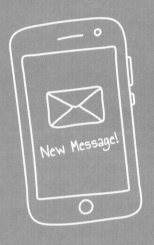

Text or email me at work to tell me how special I am to you.

#15

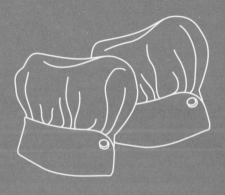

Spend an afternoon or evening **cooking** with me. Let's try to come up with our own recipe!

#16

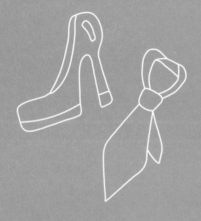

Dress up and **take me out**
to my favourite restaurant
or bar, or take me for a trip
outdoors with our own picnic.

#17

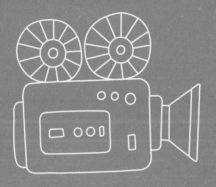

Watch a movie
(my choice) and
snuggle up under a
blanket with me.

#18

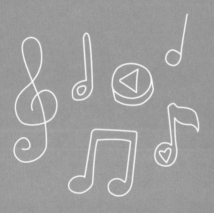

Surprise me by playing
a romantic song
and asking for a
slow dance.

#19

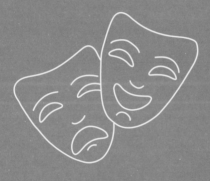

Watch a **comedy** show or funny film with me.

#20

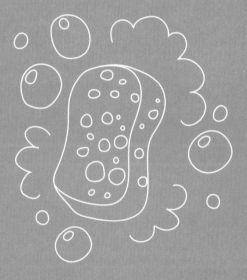

Take a **shower** with me and let's **linger** over cleaning each other.

#21

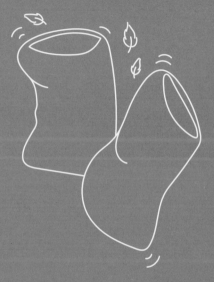

Challenge me to a pillow fight – and see where it goes...

#22

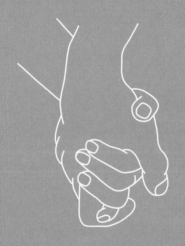

Go for a walk with
me in one of our
favourite places,
and **hold my hand.**

#23

Write down **every time you think of me** during the week, and **what you think about.** Then give me the list on the last day.

XOX

#24

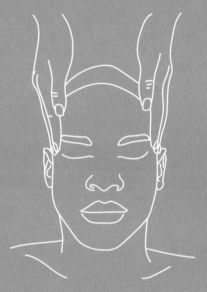

Using a gentle moisturiser, treat me to a **sensual** face massage.

#25

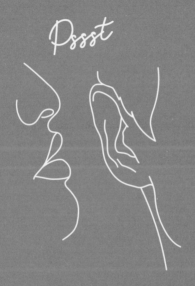

Pssst

Whisper something **romantic** to me while we're out together.

#26

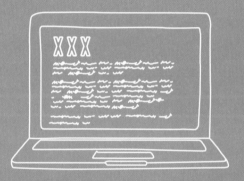

Find an erotic story online and send it to me.

#27

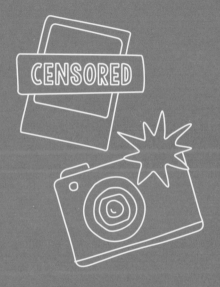

Send me a
sexy photograph
of yourself.

#28

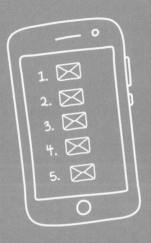

Send me five texts
during the day
describing **what
you want to do
to me tonight.**

#29

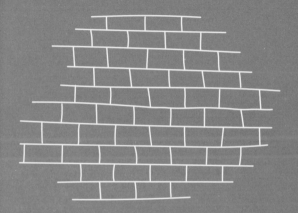

Pin me against the wall and **kiss** me or have **sex** in a **standing** position.

#30

Surprise me by pulling
me into the bedroom
as soon as I get home.

#31

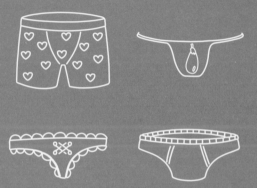

Treat me to dinner but
make sure I know you
**aren't wearing any
underwear.**

#32

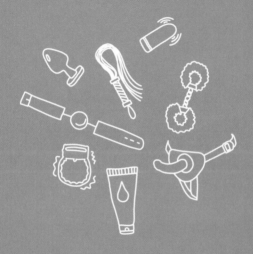

Create a sexy treasure hunt with objects that I'll be able to **use on you when I find you.**

#33

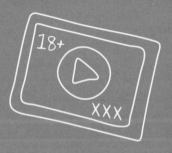

Make a sexy home
video on your own
(either **strip** or indulge
in a bit of **solo play**)
and send it to me.

#34

Strip me **naked**
and instruct me
to lie on the bed.

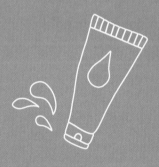

Give me an **all-over**
body massage, ending
with a **special something**
that I won't forget!

#35

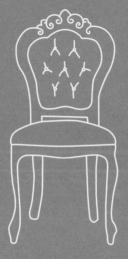

Sit me in a **chair**
and bring me to
orgasm using only
your mouth or a toy.

#36

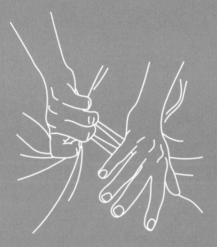

Bring me just to
the point of orgasm
however you choose...
then stop. Only finish
when I **beg.**

#37

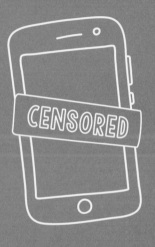

Ask me to **film** you
while you perform oral
sex on me.

#38

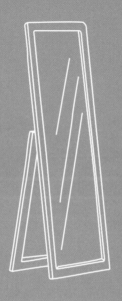

Position a mirror at
the end of our bed and
let's **watch ourselves**
making love.

#39

Pretend that you're a teacher who's caught me cheating on a test. **Discipline me** however you see fit.

#40

Make me **climax**
but tell me I have to
keep **completely quiet.**

If I make
a sound,
punish me.

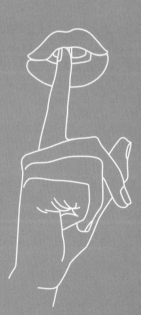

#41

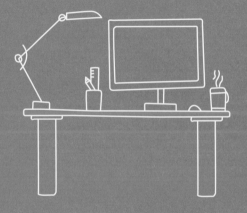

Have **sex** with me in
any room other than
the bedroom.

#42

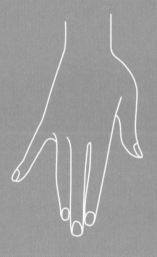

Touch yourself
while performing
oral sex on me.

#43

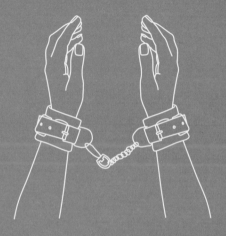

Tie my hands above my head and explore my body with your fingers and tongue.

#44

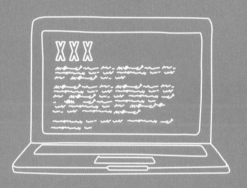

Research sex positions and try one that we've never done before.

#45

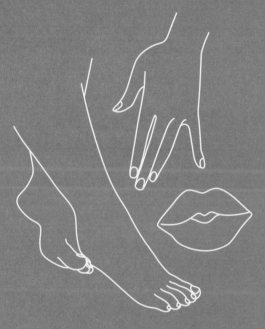

Hands, mouths, anything goes – **just no penetration.**

#46

Pretend you're a **doctor and** I'm your **patient.**

Give me an examination
I'll never forget before
administering your 'cure'.

#47

I'll write down three **fantasies**, fold them up and put them in a hat.

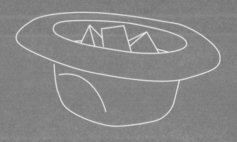

You pick one and **act it out** for me (we'll save the others for another time).

#48

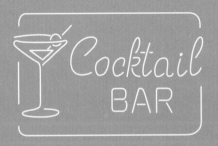

Let's go somewhere public and **pretend to be strangers.** Chat me up and take me home for a **one-night stand.**

#49

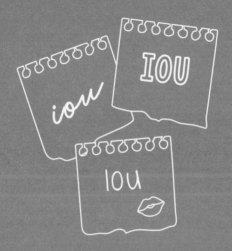

You're an escort.
Write down sexual
actions you'd be willing
to perform on me in
exchange for sexy IOUs.

#50

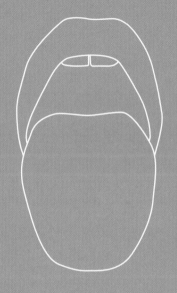

Let me **stand up** while you perform **oral sex** on me.

#51

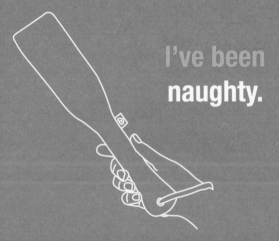

I've been **naughty.**

Pull down my underwear
and lie me over your knee.
Tell me to count as you
administer **spanks** to my
bottom with your hand
or a flat object.

#52

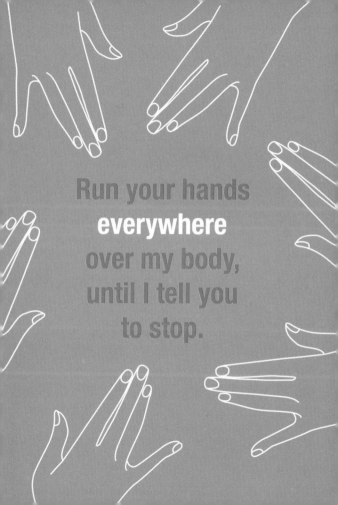

Try these out next!

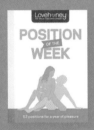

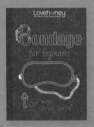

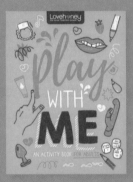

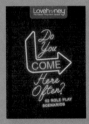

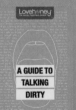